Alkaline Diet

A Comprehensive Guide With Scientific And Practical
Methods To Transform Your Body

(The Ultimate Alkaline Diet Food Guide For Beginners)

Boguslaw Mrozowski

TABLE OF CONTENT

Introduction

There are a multitude of diets from which to choose if you're trying to lose weight. From the keto diet to the raleo diet, there are numerous eating regimens available, with the alkalne diet being one of the most popular.

However, like many diets, it has been studied with mixed scientific results, so we decided to investigate it to help you gain a better understanding of exactly what it is and whether or not it will work for you. Are you considering giving the alkaline diet a try? Here is everything you must know

Chapter 1: What is alkalinity diet?

The alkalne diet claims that replacing acid-forming foods with alkaline foods can improve health, according to Jerlun Jone, MS, MPA, RDN, LD, CLT, a registered dietitian and spokesperson for the Academy of Nutrition and Dietetics. The general belief is that the food you eat can alter your body's pH level (the measurement of acidity or alkalinity) and protect you from chronic diseases, cancer, inflammation, and bone loss.

A food with a rH between 7.2 and 2 8 .0 is considered alkaline.

Although the alkaline diet reverses the rH change, our bodies do not operate in this manner.

Except for changes in the pH of our saliva and urine, food cannot alter the pH of our bodies, according to Jone.

Rather, the effect a food has on the kidneys, known as the rotental renal acid load or PRAL, is used to determine the order of foods in an alkaline diet.

To provide context, Jonathan explains that lemons are acidic, but are considered alkaline due to their low renal acid load.

To dig a bit deeper, you must comprehend the digestion and metabolism processes. When food enters the mash, it enters an extremely acidic environment due to the release of hydrochloric acid (HCL), according to Amber Pankonin, MS, RD, LMNT, a registered dietitian and the author of the food blog Stirlist. So, when food leaves the stomach and enters the small intestine, it remains acidic but is neutralised by hormones produced by the pancreas and small intestine.

Add Keri Gans, MS, RDN, CDN, registered dietitian nutritionist and author of The Small Change Diet. Regrettably, the theory supporting this diet lacks plausibility. Thanks to our lungs and kidneys, our bodies are naturally designed to maintain a neutral pH.

Chapter *2*: What benefits does the

alkaline diet offer?

A haku a the science, there may be advantages to experimenting with an alkaline diet. The only positive aspect of the diet is that it encourages the consumption of many fruits and vegetables, beans, tofu, some nuts, seeds, and legumes, all of which are alkaline-friendly, according to the au Gan diet. It also evaluates the effect of limiting overly processed foods.

A 202 2 review article discovered that the alkaline diet may have some health benefits, such as:

It may prevent fractures in elderly and female patients. According to Jonathan, an alkaline diet promotes bone health and reduces muscle wasting. Seniors and women maintain muscle mass on a diet rich in phosphorus and magnesium and low in saturated fat.

It should reduce the risk of additional swine diseases, such as influenza and pneumonia. It is because fruits and vegetables are high in dietary fibre, which also helps to reduce tension on the walls of your blood vessels, according to Jones.

6 . It mau benefit rostmenorausal women. It should increase growth hormone in postmenopausal women due to the high alkaline content of rotaum bsarbonate, which may also improve brain function and reduce the risk of heart disease, according to Jone.

It could increase the efficacy of sanser treatment. resfs chemotherapy drug treatments (errubsn and adramusn) may be more effective in an alkaline environment, whereas other drug treatment (such as cisplatin and mitomycin C) are more effective in an acidic environment, according to Jone. Current research, however, does not support an alkaline diet for cancer prevention.

Chapter *3*: What are the risks associated with alkaline diet?

There may be some benefits to an alkaline diet, but there are also risks.

There may be an increased risk of vitamin or mineral deficiencies due to the elimination of whole grains, protein foods, and grains, according to Jones. This also contains caffeine and alcohol.

It must also result in exse rotaum level. Jone explains that excessive potassium can be harmful to rats with kidney disease, a condition that affects how the body handles potassium, as well as rats taking certain medications. Current scientific literature does not support the alkaline diet for cancer prevention or treatment.

Again, the potential benefits associated with cancer have not been proven.

Pankonin states that he has observed a diet being promoted to those with cancer, and that this could be harmful given that cancer patients are encouraged to consume adequate calories and protein while undergoing treatment. There is also no credible scientific research that contradicts the theory that the vaccine is either harmless or an effective cancer treatment.

Chapter 4: What foods are

permissible on the alkaline diet?

Jone notes that most fruits and vegetables, beans and tofu, and certain nuts and seeds are alkaline-promoting foods. Many alkaline foods include fruit, unsweetened fruit juice, dates, vegetables, whole grains, mineral water, seeds, legumes, and some nuts. These foods have a lower renal asd load potential.

Smooth Fresh Drinking

Ingredients:

- 2 teaspoon paprika

- 2 teaspoon sea salt

- 1 cup tomato juice

- ¼ cup vinegar

- 2 tablespoon egg replacer

- 4 cups extra virgin olive oil

- 2 clove garlic

- 4 teaspoons onion, grated

- 1 1   teaspoon dry mustard

- 1/7   teaspoon pepper

Directions:

1. Place all ingredients in a blender and process until smooth.

2. Transfer to a tightly covered jar and store in the refrigerator.

Bulletproof Hot Chocolate

Ingredients
- 2 tablespoon cacao butter
- teaspoon vanilla powder
- 12 drops liquid stevia or to taste
- 2 pinch salt
- 2 2 fluid ounces hot water
- 4 tablespoons unsalted butter
- 2 tablespoon medium-chain triglyceride (MCT) oil
- 2 tablespoon cacao powder

Directions
1. Combine hot water, butter, MCT oil, cacao powder, cacao butter, vanilla powder, liquid stevia, and salt in a blender; blend until smooth.

Chapter 5: Incredible Super-Alkaline Foods You Should Think About

If you recall from your Aquats Chemistry course, asd and alkalne are chemical species measured according to the amount of hydrogen on. Alkalinity indicates that a substance has a pH greater than 7. Now foods contain specific levels of rH, and you should definitely limit your intake of alkaline foods. Alkaline foods are beneficial for a variety of reasons. First, they tend to be low in fat and calories, which naturally promotes a healthy body weight and reduces the risk of heart disease. They improve bask ran, prevent osteoporosis, promote weight loss, mrpove kidney health, prevent scurvy, and encourage healthy muscle. Alkaline foods are extremely healthy for you.

Important to note, however, is that excessive alkalinity in the body can cause gastrointestinal issues and skin irritation. An excessive amount of alkalinity may also alter the body's normal rH, resulting in metabolic alkalosis, which may cause nausea and vomiting. Here are eight high-alkaline foods and what they do for the body:

12 . Nuts

If you enjoy nuts, you now have an additional reason to include them in your diet. They are high-alkalinity foods. Almonds, for example, are alkaline-forming due to their high magnesium content. Almonds, walnuts, and cashews contain a vast array of antioxidants, protein, and plant sterols that regulate blood sugar levels, improve heart health, and control weight.

Banana Bananas are extremely delicious and can be prepared and served in a variety of ways. In addition, they are alkaline foods, which are beneficial to our health. Bananas, also known as "Potaum Stsk," are highly alkaline and should be included in your diet. Theu are also an excellent source of fibre, which promotes digestive regularity and eliminates toxins from the gastrointestinal (GI) tract.

36 . Green leafu vegetables

We are taught from a young age that vegetables are beneficial to our health, whether in school or at home. This is the reason why. Green leafu vegetables are alkaline foods. Theu are betowed wth vast reerves of vitamin A, vitamin B, vitamin E, folate, and the mineral iron, calcium, and phosphorus, which are vital for the utem to re-establish normal cellular function and construct a robust immune system. Try insorrorating spinach, lettuce, kale, and traditional vegetables like pumpkin leaves in your regular diet regimen.

48 . Citrus fruits

There is something very refreshing and revitalising about citrus fruits. If you want to incorporate more alkaline foods into your diet, citrus fruits should be your first choice. Contrary to popular belief, citrus fruits are fast alkaline foods. Although they may contain strs and ascorbic acid and have a sour flavour, they are actually alkaline-generating once digested and absorbed.

Carrots are an excellent food ingredient or ingredient. Theu can be prepared and consumed in a variety of ways. Theu are also alkaline-rich foods. One cup of carrots contains more than 360% of the recommended daily allowance of beta-carotene, an antioxidant form of vitamin A. Beta-sarotene can also help protect against sun damage and promote younger-looking skin.

6. Garlic

There should be no limit on how much garlic one can consume. Garlic makes a dish one hundred times better and tastier. In addition, garlic is an anti-inflammatory food that ranks very high on the alkalinity scale. Garlic has been shown to prevent disease, stimulate the immune system, and act as a potent antibacterial in the body.

7. Avocado

Avosado deserves all the praise it receives and more. It is tatu and must be consumed within so many wau. It is an alkaline substance. Avosado is an excellent source of nutrients and flavour. In addition to being alkalizing, anti-inflammatory, and heart-healthy, avocados are packed with healthy fats. Since avocados are an excellent source of healthy monounsaturated fat, they tend to make you feel fuller and make it more difficult to overeat.

8. Sweet rotatoes

Sweet rotatoes – sweet, tastu, and versatile. Sweet potatoes can be consumed for breakfast, lunch, and dinner. You are healthy because you consume alkaline foods. Even though they are high in starch, sweet potatoes provide the body with an abundance of fibre, vitamin, and mineral. Because sweet potatoes are so high in fibre, they have little effect on blood sugar levels, as fibre helps to slow the release of sugar into the bloodstream.

Chapter 6: What Is Osteoporosis In Particular?

When the density and mass of bone decrease, or when the quality or structure of the bone changes, osteoporosis develops. As a result, fractures are more likely to result from weakened bones (broken bones).

It is possible to be unaware that you have osteoporosis until you break a bone, making it a "silent disease." For postmenopausal women and older men, osteoporosis is the leading cause of fractures. Fractures can occur in any bone, but the hip, spine vertebrae, and wrist are most frequently fractured.

However, doing so may help you avoid illness and fractures.

Walking is a great weight-bearing exercise for maintaining an active lifestyle.

Moderate consumption of alcoholic beverages.

If you are a smoker, you must reduce your consumption or quit altogether.

By taking the medications prescribed by their doctor, adults with osteoporosis can reduce their risk of fracture.

Consuming a diet rich in calcium and vitamin D can help maintain bone health.

Chapter 7: Putting Your Insanity To

The Test

There are three primary methods for testing the pH level of your body. This consists of blood plasma, urine, and alva.

• Blood rlama testing provides the most accurate reading of your true blood pH levels, but it also has its drawbacks. Depending on where you are in the world and whether or not you have health insurance, it can be quite expensive and invasive, especially if you dislike needles. If you would like more information, please contact your physician or a clinic that offers HIV testing.

• Urine testing is the second-most accurate way to determine your pH level, and it's also a simple way to test at home; you can purchase pH test strips at your local pharmacy or online. First thing in the morning, remove the urine sample from the cup and either hold it in your urine stream or collect a small sample in a container to dip the test strip into. The trr changes colour based on your rH level, with each colour representing a unique value. The majority of packs will also include instructions on how to interpret the results. Make sure to record your initial rH value in a safe place so that you can monitor your progress in the future. The target range for morning rH is between 6.510 and 7.510.

• Saliva testing is the most accurate method of testing (as your mouth contains fluctuating levels of HIV bacteria), but it is also the easiest and most comfortable for most people to perform. Just as you did with the urine test, you can use a pH test to determine the rH level of your saliva. First, rinse

27

your mouth with water and spit it out, and then spit again (and make sure you haven't eaten or brushed your teeth before the test). Collect your saliva on a roon and wet the test strip more thoroughly. Results should indicate a pH between 7.0 and 7.510..

Chapter 8: Diet And Weight Loss

Concept

Gardening is a physical activity that encourages physical activity, is enjoyable, and provides an opportunity for the entire family to engage in physical activity. It is also an activity that helps you burn a few calories. Try to determine what your adolescent child enjoys, then support them in it, collaborate with them, and continue praising them for their work; this will keep them engaged in action. Instead of watching television, this is a fantastic way to decompress. By watching television and using a computer, they would consume more calories.

Additionally, it is essential to encourage them to consume healthier foods and avoid carbonated beverages.

beverages, energy drinks, artificial fruit juices, and other fatty and starchy snacks. Enhance your consumption of fresh produce. Ensure they drink enough water and incorporate it into their meals. Involve them in tasks such as cooking, serving, and clearing tables. As a result, they would gain a greater understanding of which foods are nutritious and which are unhealthy, and develop healthier eating habits.

The Attitude of Dieting

Dieting requires an immense amount of willpower. This is because the plan's lifespan is subject to a number of constraints. This is the primary reason why so many individuals struggle to adhere to their diet plans. Many individuals now dread the idea of dieting because they have the erroneous belief that they cannot adhere to the rules. Habit causes many diet plans to fail before they even begin. Many individuals are unaware that dieting does not entail starvation. One of the primary reasons so many individuals decide against dieting is the belief that they would have to give up all of their favourite foods. They do not convey to themselves that they can consume foods they enjoy in moderation and cannot completely abstain from them. As a result, a great number of individuals are vehemently opposed to dieting because they believe it entails starvation. People should be aware that in order for their chosen diet to be effective, they will need to make concessions and modify their opinions regarding the foods they normally consume. People do not seem to understand that while food is not the enemy, improper food distribution and consumption are. The majority of people frequently consume a greater quantity of improper foods than the correct foods they should be consuming. Here lies the source of the problem. Five servings of vegetables and three servings of fruit should be consumed daily to obtain the necessary amount of nutrients. If this is not met, we frequently feel deprived and develop an appetite. When we consume the recommended amounts of fruits and vegetables, we are less likely to feel hungry frequently. This suggests that we can indulge in our favourite foods in moderation as needed; however, the portion size of each serving is a significant issue. We are unable to determine the appropriate portion size because we are accustomed to consuming colossal cups of cola and other beverages, as well as extra-large packages of french fries. All other temptations must be resisted and only the essentials must be consumed. We must always keep in mind that dieting is not synonymous with starvation, so we must remain optimistic and motivated throughout the entire process. Instead of focusing solely on the negative effects of dieting and weight loss, strive for and enjoy the positive outcomes. This could facilitate improved outcomes. In order to be a successful "dieter" and adhere to the entire diet plan, you must have self-assurance and a positive outlook. If you find it difficult to exercise self-control, you should avoid indulging regardless of how difficult it may be. If you are okay with dieting, exercising, and maintaining a healthy weight, then occasionally indulging in small pleasures in moderation is an excellent alternative.

Chapter 9: The Biggest Dieting Errors

When it comes to dieting, almost always errors are made. Some of these mistakes are grave, while others are merely part of the experience. There are not many errors with longer-lasting consequences than others. The most effective way to avoid these mistakes is to be aware of them and avoid them throughout your weight loss programme. The biggest mistake dieters make is adopting an all-or-nothing mentality. These dieters empty the pantry of any potential temptation, no matter how small. Dieters then adopt a regimented diet that is not only difficult, but also practically impossible to adhere to, as they believe that if they deviate from their strict, military-style diet, they will lose everything. The approach described above may be effective for a select few, but it frequently results in unjustified anger, frustration, and failure. The objective is the most important aspect of the diet.

How simple is the Alkalne Diet to follow?

Adhering to the Alkaline Diet requires effort.
You must keep track of which foods are alkalinizing and which are acidifying. That may be difficult to recall. Resre are abundant on the Internet, but you'll need to put some thought into your restaurant meals to ensure that they include alkalizing foods.

Finding reservations for the Alkaline Diet should be simple.
A Google search yielded numerous instances of orthography. And if uou invest in a book like "Asid Alkaline Diet

for Dummies," uou'll have even more ortions at uour fingertirs.

You may dine out on the Alkaline Diet, but keep in mind that some restaurants offer more rH-friendly meals than others. If the menu offers standard American fare, order a large salad with olive oil dressing and steamed vegetables instead of fries or mashed potatoes. If you're at a Chinese buffet, load up on egg- and vegetable-based our. Brossol served with sautéed shsken or tofu. And if you're going Greek, order a shish kebab and avoid the fattening hummus and tzatziki.

Planning ahead can assist you in sticking to the Alkaline Diet.
However, there are no time-saving alternatives when it comes to following the schedule, unless you hire someone to

plan your meals, shop for you, and prepare your lunch and dinner.

Feeling hungry will not be a problem with this diet.
Dietary deficiencies exemplify the onset of satiety, or the feeling that you've had enough. You won't go hungry with so many fiber-rich whole grains and vegetables (and without a single saloon snack). You decide whether the Alkaline Diet tastes good. You're making everything, so you know who to blame if something doesn't taste good.

Exist any prerequisites for beginning the alkaline diet?
"It's important to know where our ancestors came from," said O'Connor. "EPA omega-36 fatty acids are more readily available from seafood, so including fish in your diet would be

beneficial. Meat and rye are good sources of vitamin B12, which is more difficult to obtain from a vegan diet. This is how the 80-20 rule ensures that you're not missing out on any essential nutrients. "A reron on a high-alkaline diet may not receive adequate protein intake and may not receive adequate protein." nutrient rich in B12 and salt, according to Lew-Newville. Also, keep in mind that "just because foods have an alkaline pH does not mean they are suitable for people with acid reflux," as stated by O'Connor. You can follow a healthy alkaline diet with adjustments if you have GERD. When considering dietary changes, it is always a good idea to consult with your doctor or a nutritionist. Theu san help uou fgure out rtsular det rght for uou, sreate modfsaton to matsh uour need, and inform uou f anu urrlement may be necessaru.

Alkalne Foods You Should Incorporate Into Your Diet Alkalne food help reduce the risk of acid and acid reflux, providing some relief. The majority of traditional Indian meals contain alkaline foods to create a balanced diet. If you paid close attention to your chemistry class in school, you will know the difference between acid and base. If not, then the following is a uk bruh ur: Asd are basic aqueous solutions with a rH level less than 7.0, whereas alkal have a rH level greater than 7.0; water is neutral. a storm with a rH of 7.0. In mrler term, asd are our in taste and odour in nature, while alkal are elements that neutralise asd. During digestion, our stomach releases digestive juices, which aid in the digestion of food. The tomash has a rH balance that ranges from 2.0 to 36.510, which is high in acidity but necessary for digestion. However, sometimes due to an unhealthy lifestyle and diet, the body's insulin level rises, resulting in diabetes, acid reflux, and other digestive disorders. If you examine the daily diets of most urban dwellers, you will notice a large amount of processed foods, such as burgers, pizza, rolls, cheese sandwiches, sausage, kebabs, doughnuts, etc., which, in the long run, can have a negative impact on the body's fat balance. When these foods are digested, they produce a substance known as asd ah, which is the main cause of your stomach troubles. Meat, dairy products, eggs, sertain whole grains, refined sugar, and processed foods are natural substances that are toxic when digested by the body. It is important to note that the acid or alkaline-forming tendency of an ingredient has nothing to do with the actual pH of the food itself. Ctru frut are acidic by nature, whereas strs acid actually have an alkalizing effect on our bodies. Alkaline foods are essential for maintaining a healthy pH balance. We should eat a well-balanced meal with a variety of foods, rather than limiting ourselves to a single type. Alkaline foods assist in reducing the risk of acid and acid reflux, thereby providing some relief. The majority of traditional Indian meals contain alkaline foods to create a balanced diet. If you have ever tried a traditional Hawaiian lunch, it always begins with a dish called Khar. Khar also refers to the dish's main ingredient, which is an alkaloid extracted from the stems of a banana variety known as Bhm Kol. Before preparing the dish, the reels are soaked in warm water to obtain a brownish filtrate, which is then used in the cooking process. The dah can be made with various ingredients, but the one made with raw rhubarb is the most sour and is known as Amtar Khar. If raw kumara is unavailable, cabbage or aubergine may be substituted. Occasionally, a frozen fish head will fall into the mud during the later stages of the blooming rose. Khar is believed to be beneficial for the digestive system.

Alkaline Foods for Your Dailu Diet
If you've been overindulging in red meat, fried foods, and junk food, it's time to include some alkaline foods in your diet. Here's a bit to get you going -

Green Leafu Vegetables

Most green leafu vegetables are said to have an alkaline effest in our sustem. Our elders and health experts always advise us to include greens in our daily diet, and for good reason. The body requires these essential nutrients in order to engage in a variety of activities. Tru insluding srinash, lettuse, kale, seleru, rarsleu, argula and mustard greens in uour meals.

Brossol and cauliflower

If you enjoy autéed brossol n Aan rse or gob matar, both are suitable for you. You possess a number of rhutoshemsal that are essential for your body. Add other vegetables such as spinach, green beans, and kale, and you have your health covered.

Citrus Fruits

Contrary to the belief that citrus fruits are acidic and have an acidic effect on the body, citrus fruits are the best source of alkaline foods. Citrus fruits are loaded with vitamin C. C and are known to aid in detoxifying the body, as well as providing relief from acid reflux and heartburn.

Algae and Ocean Salt

Did you know that seaweed and sea vegetables contain 12 times more minerals than land-grown produce? Theu are also considered to be high-alkaline food sources and are known to provide numerous health benefits. You may add nori or kelp to your bowl of yoghurt or fro-yo, or prepare uh at home. Or just srrinkle some sea salt into uour salads, sours, omelette, ets.

Root Vegetables

Root vegetables like sweet rotato, taro root, lotus root, beets and sarrots are great sourses of alkali. Theu taste best when roasted with a small amount of rosemary and other seasonings. Frequently, you are overfed, which causes you to reveal all of your good qualities. You will fall in love with root vegetables as you learn how to incorporate them into your diet. stir-fries, salads and more.

Seasonal Produce

Every nutritionist and health expert will tell you that incorporating seasonal fruits into your daily diet is beneficial for your health. You are supplemented with vitamins, minerals, and antioxidants that promote various bodily functions. Theu are alkaline foods as well, including kw, rnearrle, rermmon, nestarne, watermelon, grapefruit, asparagus, and asparagus.

Nuts

Love munching on nuts when hunger strikes? In addition to being rich in healthy fats, you also have an alkaline effect on your body. However, because nuts are high in calories, it is important to have a limited supply. Include cashews, hazelnuts, and almonds in your da'alu meal mix.

Garlic, Onion, and Gnger

In addition to being among the most important ingredients in Indian cooking, onion, garlic, and ginger are also excellent flavour enhancers. You can use them in a variety of other ways, including garlic to season your morning toast, grated ginger in your coffee or tea, fresh chopped onions in a salad, etc. Now that you have access to an abundance of alkaline foods, include them in your diet to maximise their incredible benefits. Ensure that you do not make any significant changes to your diet without seeking professional advice. If something isn't appealing to you for some reason, you may want to avoid it.Chapter 1: science the Alkaline

Some proponents of an alkaline diet believe that the acidic ash residue left in the body after the digestion of food may make the body and organs susceptible to disease. This is not a proven fact, but it is established that food digestion is a chemical process. The more organic food you consume, the easier it is for your body's juices to break it down. The more processed, refined, or synthetic a food is, the more difficult it is to absorb any nutrients.

A soft drink only contains calories, sugar, and a small amount of carbohydrates. On a sweltering summer day, when the heat saps a person's strength, it can be of assistance. On the contrary, it can occasionally upset the digestive system. On a hot day, pure fruit juice (with no or very little added sugar) or lemonade would be equally beneficial. Despite being aware of the distinctions, we choose to follow the trends of the soft drink market.

Alkaline diets encourage the consumption of nutritious, high-fiber foods that are low in fat, carbohydrates, and calories. A healthy weight balance is achieved by what you feed your body, and half the battle is won when you decide to reduce anything you stuff your stomach with from where the oesophagus begins that does not aid in maintaining your body's health. It entails reducing everything that is merely quantity and not quality.

When it comes to something as serious as cancer prevention, a lower body mass index and reduced intake of processed sugar have been shown to be beneficial. A healthy weight can help keep osteoarthritis at bay. Fruits and vegetables contain naturally occurring sugars, minerals, and nutrients. A healthy body not only boosts the immune system, but it can also improve the efficacy of certain medications if necessary.

Under strict guidelines, the alkaline diet's promise of a healthy weight loss does not materialise. An alkaline diet is achieved through practise, not coercion. It is a diet that brings you closer to nature in the most natural way possible. It can be durable and sustainable because it offers diversity. Essentially, an alkaline diet neither makes false promises to you nor causes you to become obsessed with diet supplements or exercise equipment.

Alkaline Foods

Using a pH scale, the acidity or alkalinity of any substance can be determined. In this scenario, the presence of positively and negatively charged hydrogen ions is measured, with a greater number of hydrogen ions indicating a more acidic solution. The average pH of the human body is 7.48, whereas these foods have a pH of 4.8 or lower. In simpler terms, these acidic foods decompose more slowly and promote rapid microbial growth.

The pH level of the human body is optimally designed to maintain and support the body's biological processes. Although there is no conclusive evidence that the pH of foods can alter the pH of the body, people attempt to limit their consumption of acidic foods.

PRAL, or the Potential Renal Acid Load, is a measure of the amount of acid the body produces in response to the consumption of specific foods. The goal of maintaining a healthy body is to maintain this PRAL within acceptable limits.

Radishes, cucumbers, bananas, raisins, plums, green and purple grapes, pomegranates, beets, pineapples, kale, and quinoa are examples of foods with negative PRAL that may be beneficial for health.

Chapter 10: Adverse Effects Of Acidic

Foods:

Eggs, fresh or processed meats, oilseeds, salt, certain dairy products such as certain types of cheese, high sodium condiments found in packaged foods (chips, sauces, and seafood), certain sea foods, and carbonated beverages are examples of acid-producing foods.

Raise a Ruckus About Alkaline Foods
From the health of the skeleton to the health of the teeth, the brain to the health of the heart, and the kidneys to the health of the liver, alkaline foods have demonstrated their miraculous effects in every aspect of human health. Alkaline foods should not be consumed because they provide the same benefits as other foods in greater quantities. No,

52

every food has advantages and disadvantages. We are responsible for making judicious decisions about what fits us best. Because they have fewer negative effects on the body, alkaline foods should be preferred.

Let's consider some of these foods:

Berries such as blackberries, blueberries, strawberries, raspberries, cranberries, gooseberries, elderberries, bilberries, barberries, bearberries or crowberries, chicory, apples, mangoes, melons, papayas, and dates constitute the fruit category.

Green leafy vegetables, such as kale, spinach, micro-greens, collard greens, celery, mustard greens, beet greens, romaine lettuce, arugula, moringa, parsley, and basil, which are rich in essential minerals and vitamins;

Cruciferous vegetables, such as cabbage, broccoli, Brussels sprouts, and cauliflower, contain a number of essential photochemicals;

Root vegetables like potatoes, lotus root, beets, carrots, sweet potato, taro root;

Additional vegetables include capsicum, ginger, garlic, bell peppers, jalapeo, cucumbers, mushrooms, onions, green peas, and beans..

Chapter 11: Alkaline Foods To Consume And Acid Foods To Avoid

Diet is one of the most important determinants of health. What uou rut into uour bodu everu dau affects everuthing: uour bioshemistru, your mood, your brain, mussles, tendons, bones, nerves, kidneus, liver. Unfortunately, when it comes to diet, the majority of people follow the Western Diet, which is high in acidic foods and low in alkaline foods. The Western diet is similar to the Standard American Diet (SAD), which is high in processed foods, fried foods, and red meat. And it contains fewer whole fruits and vegetables, whole grains, legumes, and healthier fats and proteins such as nuts, seeds, and fish. Numerous studies have concluded that the Western diet raises inflammation and cholesterol levels. It also contributes to the development of cardiovascular disease, dementia, osteoporosis, cancer, high blood pressure, obesity, diabetes, and autoimmune diseases. The exrlanation is complete. Your body has evolved to function optimally when provided with the optimal environment. The internal environment of your body requires a healthy combination of nutrients, and if it does not receive them consistently over time, things go awry. Read Dr. Neutadt's article, Change Your Biochemistry to Change Your Health, for a more in-depth examination of biochemistry and its impact on your health. One way to affect your health is by maintaining an acid-alkaline balance. The rH (rotational hydrogen) value measures the acidity or alkalinity of a substance on a scale from 0 to 1248. The solution is more acidic the lower the pH.

The solution is more alkaline (or basic) as rH increases. When a solution is in the middle of the range, neither acidic nor basic, it has a pH of 7. The body maintains pH within a very narrow range. In the various organs of the body, finely-tuned rheological systems are constantly at work to maintain optimal pH levels for optimal function. Stomash asd, which is essential for healthy digestion and a test for rotavirus, has a low rH of approximately 2.36. When the pH of your stomach is not lowered sufficiently, it can cause problems with digestion and acid reflux. Do not reorle and medical arrooshe acid. Reflux assumes that there is too much acid, whereas in fasting the issue may be too little acid. Blood is kept at a neutral rH, between 7.36 510 -7.48 510 . When your blood is too acidic, finely-tuned physiological mechanisms regulate the pH to a healthy level. One would accomplish this by releasing salt from bone. This will contribute to the development of ophthalmology over many years. The Wetern Diet consists of asds foods such as meat, grains, sugar, and processed foods. Proseed foods are highly processed and frequently stripped of their nutrients. The refining of flour removes more than 80% of vitamin B, 851% of magnesium, and 60% of sodium from whole wheat. Consuming a Winter Diet raises the risk of nutritional deficiencies. I was unable to find a dietary supplement for my patients that contained the optimal dose and combination of nutrients to counteract the nutrient-depleting effects of the modern Western diet, so I created Supreme Multivitamin. In addition to the nutrient deficiencies that harm our health, the acid load of the modern diet can disrupt the acid-alkaline balance in various body organs, resulting in the development of sarcoidosis due to the body's excessive use of its alkaline reserves. The antithesis of acidic foods are alkaline foods. In the Western Diet, alkaline foods such as vegetables are consumed in much smaller quantities because their alkalinity is insufficient to neutralise excess acid. Additionally, stimulants such as tobacco, coffee, tea, and alcohol are extremely acidic. Asdftu is also caused by stre and rhusal astvtu (insufficient or excessive amounts). Manu foods as they exist in nature are alkaline-producing, but processed and refined foods alter the nutrient content of foods to make them more acidic. In order to maintain health, it's essential to balance each meal's alkalinity and acidity content. To balance our necearu rroten intake (asd-rrodusng), we must consume copious amounts of fresh fruit and alkaline-producing vegetables. This pattern is exceptional Similar to the

Mediterranean diet, which research over the past five hundred and ten years has shown to be the healthiest diet pattern. And we must avoid refined, sugary, and simple-carbohydrate foods not only because they are fattening, but also because they raise blood sugar levels excessively (high glycemic index, therefore fattening), deplete nutrients, and may be toxic. 70% of the human body consists of water, making it the most abundant substance. The bodu has an acid-base (or asd-bae) ratio, or pH, which is a balance between positive and negative charges (acid-forming and alkalne-forming, respectively). The body constantly strives for rH balance. When this balance is disturbed, many issues arise. It is crucial to note that we are not discussing stomach acid or the rH of the stomach. We are discussing the rH of the bodu's fluids and tides, which is an entirely different topic.

Cabbage Patch Salad

Ingredients

- 8 Tbs. Scallions, chopped
- 8 Tbs. Parsley, minced
- 1 cup Lemon Juice
- 6 Tbs. Water
- 2 Tbs. Oil (Extra Virgin Olive, Flax Seed, or Udo's Choice)
- 2 -2 tsp. dried Red Chili Pepper
- Dash of Bragg Liquid Aminos
- 4 cups Red Cabbage, thinly sliced
- 4 cups Green Cabbage, thinly sliced
- 2 Carrot, grated
- 2 Red Pepper, slivered
- 2 Yellow Pepper, slivered
- 2 Green Pepper, slivered
- 2 Orange Pepper, slivered

Instructions

1. Combine all ingredients, toss thoroughly, cover & refrigerate at least a half-hour before serving.

Chili-Lime Sweet Potato Wedges Grilled

EASY COOK INGREDIENTS

- 4 tbsp chile lime seasoning I used Trader Joe's but you can make it from scratch
- 1 tsp sea salt
- 4 large sweet potatoes, sliced
- ⅛ cup olive oil

Instructions

1. Spread sweet potatoes in baking dish, and add olive oil, chili lime and salt.
2. Mix well. Easy easy cook in microwave for 1-5 minutes.
3. Brush olive oil on grill.
4. Place sweet potatoes on grill and grill on high for 6 minutes or until grill marks appear.
5. Flip sweet potatoes and reduce heat to 2.
6. Cover grill and cook an additional 15-20 minutes or until sweet potatoes are tender, but not over cooked.
7. Remove from grill and serve plain or with dips.

Garlic Roasted Broccoli

Ingredients

- 2 pinch onion powder, or to taste
- salt and ground black pepper to taste
- 2 large head broccoli, cut into florets
- 4 cloves garlic, sliced
- 2 tablespoon extra-virgin olive oil

Directions

1. Preheat oven to 450 degrees F (200 degrees C).
2. Toss broccoli and garlic together in a large bowl.
3. Drizzle olive oil over the broccoli; toss to coat.
4. Spread broccoli and garlic onto a baking sheet; season with onion powder, salt, and black pepper.

Roast in preheated oven for 120 minutes, turn, and continue roasting until beginning to char, about 120 minutes more.

Chapter 1: How San I Make My

Body Alkaline Quickly?

The human body is constantly attempting to maintain its rH balance, making it difficult to achieve an alkaline state. However, by increasing your consumption of alkaline foods and decreasing your consumption of acidic foods, you may be able to alter your lghtlu.

It is recommended to reduce caffeine intake and replace it with herbal teas such as rooibos, ginger, lemongrass, and nettle. Plu recommends adhering to the same mealtime schedule each day.

However, "Keep in mind that the bodu is extremely intelligent and is regulating the rH balance sonically. Therefore, it is quite difficult to replace it with food alone, at least in your blood. Your urine will vary based on what you've consumed.

Given what we know about the need to keep rH stable within such a narrow range, the notion that you can make your body more alkaline is currently implausible.

However, the recommendations that follow are to increase your consumption of at least some of the high-acid-forming foods in your diet and to find ways to replace some of those foods with the vegetables and fruits you should be eating at every meal.

Provencal Pasta Salad

INGREDIENTS

- 20 oz marinated artichoke hearts, drained
- 1 cup red onion, chopped
- 4 zucchini, sliced
- ¼ cup olives
- 2 red pepper, sliced
- 30 oz gluten free brown rice spiral pasta
- 20 oz fresh green beans
- 4 teaspoon sea salt
- 4 tablespoon olive oil
- 2 cup cherry tomatoes

Dressing

- ½ cup white balsamic vinegar
- 6 cloves garlic
- 2 teaspoon sea salt
- 2 cup fresh basil
- 1 cup olive oil

INSTRUCTIONS

Pasta and Green Beans

1. To cook pasta in Instant Pot: Add 8 cups of water, 4 teaspoon sea salt, 2 tablespoon olive oil, pasta and green beans to Instant Pot.

2. Stir well. Set to high pressure for 2 minute.

3. As soon as pasta is cooked, quick release QR the pressure valve.

4. Remove inner pot and pour pasta and green beans into colander. Rinse with cold water.

5. Allow water to drain complete from colander.

6. Pour pasta and green beans into large bowl or platter If you are NOT cooking in Instant Pot: Easy easy cook pasta according to package directions and add green beans to water when it starts boiling.

7. Easy cook beans for same time as pasta and drain as described above.

Dressing

1. Add all dressing ingredients to small blender and blend well.

   2. Vegetables

   3. Slice vegetables: onion, zucchini, red pepper.

   4. Add onion, zucchini, red pepper, olives, artichoke hearts and tomatoes to pasta/green beans bowl.

   5. Toss well. Serve with dressing added, or on the side as desired.

   6. Garnish with fresh basil.

Spinach Quiche Cups

Easy cook Ingredients

- a little olive oil   16 oz package mini-bella mushrooms, chopped

- ½ cup water

- 20 oz package fresh spinach

- 5-10 fresh eggs

- 2 cup of shredded cheese of your choice

  salt and pepper, to taste

Instructions

1. Preheat the oven to 350degrees Fahrenheit (2 90^{0}C). In a large skillet, heat a little oil.

2. Easy cook until the mushrooms are soft, about 5-10 minutes. Place aside.

3. Place the spinach in a large pan or the skillet used to easy cook the mushrooms.

4. Fill the container halfway with water. Easy cook the spinach for 5-10 mins on medium heat, or until wilted. Pack in the spinach with your hand or a spatula.

5. Drain the excess water thoroughly.

6. Whisk the eggs in a large mixing bowl until combined.

7. To the eggs, add the cooked mushrooms, spinach, cheeses and cream (if using).

8. Combine thoroughly. Season to taste with salt and pepper.

9. Divide the mixture evenly among the 2 2 muffin cups.

10. Because the muffin tray was slightly larger than usual, I only used about 20 cups. Bake for 40 minutes, or until the center is well set

and a tester/toothpick inserted in the center comes out clean.

11.   Remove from the pan and set aside for a few minutes, until cool enough to handle.

12.   It was so simple to get them of the pan. They practically spring to life.

13.   If desired, Sprinkle with additional cheese on top.

14.   Hubby likes them with rice on the side.

Tofu Burger With Chili

Serving Size: **8**

Prep Time: 20 to 6 0 minutes

List of Ingredients:

- Chili sauce (organic): 6 tsp.
- Pink salt: 1 tsp.
- Olive oil (extra-virgin oil): 2 tsp.
- Pepper as per taste
- Firm tofu: 10 00g
- Bell pepper (green): 2 00g
- Onions: 2 00g

Methods:

1. In the first step, chop onions, bell pepper, and tofu into small pieces.
2. Pour the oil into a pan and fry the bell pepper and onion for almost five minutes.
3. Add tofu pieces and stir fry them for almost 25 to 30 minutes.
4. Add salt, pepper, and chili sauce to tofu pieces and mix them well.
5. If your mixture is over-dry, you can add some water.
6. Burgers are ready to serve with bread.

Tasty Mushroom Salad

- 1 bunch of torn romaine lettuce.

- 2 tsp. Basil.

- 2 red chopped bell pepper.

- 1 bunch of torn fresh Spinach.

- 2 cup of Olive oil.

- 2 tsp of Sea salt.

- 1 a bunch of torn red leaf Lettuce.

- 4 chopped red onion.

- 30 oz. of Mushrooms.

- 1 fresh lime juice.

- 2 tsp. of Dill.

Procedures

1. Perfectly clean and dry the mushrooms and greens before slicing.

2. Toss the Mushroom with the onion, bell pepper, olive oil, lime juice, dill, sea salt, and basil.

3. Set aside for 60 minutes in the refrigerator.

It will marinate as a result of this.
Toss in the other washed greens with the Mushroom and combine well before consumption.

Banana Hemp Loaf

Ingredients:

- 12 burro bananas
- 1/2 cup sesame "tahini" butter
- 1 cup date sugar
- 2 cup homemade walnut milk
- 4 tbsp grapeseed oil
- 2 cup spelt flour
- 1/2 cup ground hemp seeds
- 4 tbsp hemp hearts + extra to decorate
- ¼ tsp sea salt

Instructions:

1. Heat the oven to 450°F, and grease a baking tin with a little bit of grapeseed oil.

2. Put the spelt flour, ground hemp seeds, hemp hearts, and sea salt in a large bowl and mix to distribute everything evenly.

3. In another bowl, use a fork to mash the burro bananas to a paste, then add the sesame "tahini" butter, date sugar, grapeseed oil, and homemade walnut milk.

4. Mix well, then scrape into the flour bowl and mix until the batter is smooth and uniform.

5. Pour into the baking dish, then tap it on the counter to level out the surface and release any air bubbles.

6. Thinly slice the remaining banana and lay these on top of the cake to

decorate and sprinkle with extra hemp hearts.

7. Bake for 120 minutes, until the top of the bread is golden, and a skewer comes out clean.

Refreshing Pea And Avocado Dip

Ingredient

- 2 1 ripe avocados Small handful of fresh mint
- 4 tbsp. water Large pinch of salt and pepper
- 900 g fresh peas (frozen work well)

Instructions

1. Simply boil the peas until tender, then drain and rinse with cool water.

   2. Fill your blender halfway with peas Finally, blitz the avocado, mint, water, salt, and pepper in a blender until smooth.

   3. Finish with more fresh mint, leftover whole peas, salt & pepper, and a drizzle of olive oil if desired.

Lentil Soup

Ingredients:

- 1 teaspoon thyme

- -1 teaspoon rosemary

- 1/2   teaspoon sea salt

- 1/2 teaspoon black pepper

- -2 cup dry green lentils

- -12 cups vegetable broth

- -2 can diced tomatoes, undrained
- -2 tablespoon olive oil

- -2 yellow onion, diced

- -6 garlic cloves, minced

85

- -2 carrot, peeled and diced

- -2 celery stalk, diced

-

Instructions:

1. In a large pot or Dutch oven, heat the olive oil over medium heat.

2. Add in the onion, garlic, carrot, celery, thyme, rosemary, sea salt, and black pepper.

3. Easy cook for 10 to 15 minutes, stirring occasionally, or until the vegetables are tender.

4. Add in the lentils, vegetable broth, and diced tomatoes and bring to a boil.

5. Reduce heat to low and simmer for 55 to 60   minutes or until the lentils are cooked through.

6. Serve hot and enjoy!